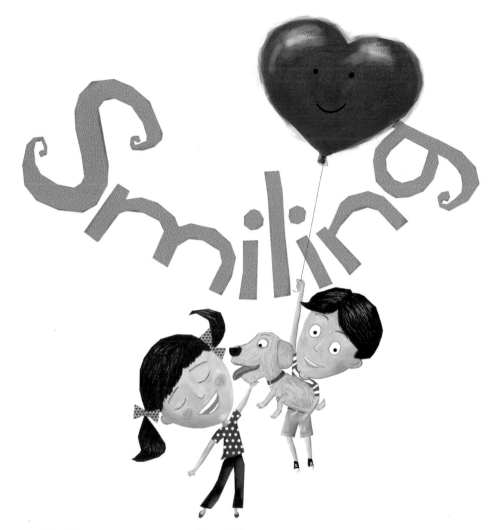

Smiling Heart Meditations

with **Lisa & Ted** (and Bingo)

Written and Illustrated by Lisa Spillane

First published in 2015
by Singing Dragon
an imprint of Jessica Kingsley Publishers
73 Collier Street
London N1 9BE, UK
and
400 Market Street, Suite 400
Philadelphia, PA 19106, USA

www.singingdragon.com

Library of Congress Cataloging in Publication Data
Spillane, Lisa, author, illustrator.
  Smiling heart meditations with Lisa and Ted (and Bingo) / Lisa Spillane.
     pages cm
   ISBN 978-1-84819-200-3 (alk. paper)
 [1. Qi gong--Fiction. 2. Meditation--Fiction.] I. Title.
  PZ7.S75476Sm 2014
  [E]--dc23
                            2014021219

British Library Cataloguing in Publication Data
A CIP catalogue record for this book is available from the British Library

ISBN 978 1 84819 200 3
eISBN 978 0 85701 168 8

Printed and bound in China

For my husband Eamon,
who makes my heart smile.
xxx

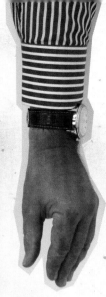

A Note for the Big People

Lisa and Ted (and Bingo too) show children how Smiling Heart Meditations can help them to let go of their impatient and resentful feelings. The techniques they demonstrate in this story were developed thousands of years ago in China to help people to release excess negative emotions from their bodies. The healing power of smiling along with sound-making and deep-breathing are combined with gentle movements and visualizations to restore calmness to the body and mind.

Put simply, they work because:

* smiling, even when you don't feel like it, stimulates a chemical reaction in your body that reduces stress and supports your immune system

* visualizing lowers cortisol and lifts your mood

* thinking kind and grateful thoughts produces chemicals that calm your nervous system, protect your heart and encourage you to think more insightfully

* and, in addition to having a calming effect, deep-breathing increases oxygen-rich blood in your body, which is needed for energy and healing. Deep-breathing and raising your arms also boosts your lymphatic system, helping it to get rid of toxins.

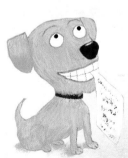

When you're doing Smiling Heart Meditations remember to breathe deeply. Allow your belly to rise as you breathe in and use your tummy muscles to gently bring it back in as you breathe out. The meditations work best if they're done in the correct order along with the other five Healing Sounds Meditations but they're also very effective when practised on their own.

I hope this book brings you and the children you share it with more patience, love and smiles, especially when you need them the most!

Patting my head, Lisa said, "I'm going to build sand-castles and swim in the sea..."

"And..?" asked Ted. "Go Skimboarding!" they screamed.

"What are you going to do, Bingo?" asked Lisa.

"Ruff, ruff!" I replied, thinking, "Play fetch!"

"Yes, you love digging in the sand," said Lisa, rubbing my ears.

You know, there are many things that people can do better than dogs, but mind-reading is certainly not one of them. Most of the time, I know what Lisa and Ted are thinking, even when we're not together. Like, I always know when they're coming home or planning to take me for a walk.

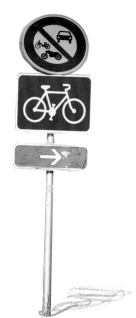

The next time I barked, I thought "doggy biscuit" with all of my brain power. Then, to make it easier for her, I licked my lips. "Later. But only if you don't jump out of the basket to run after rabbits," she warned. "Hmmm, I was looking forward to a bit of bunny-chasing... Lisa's mind-reading is improving," I thought.

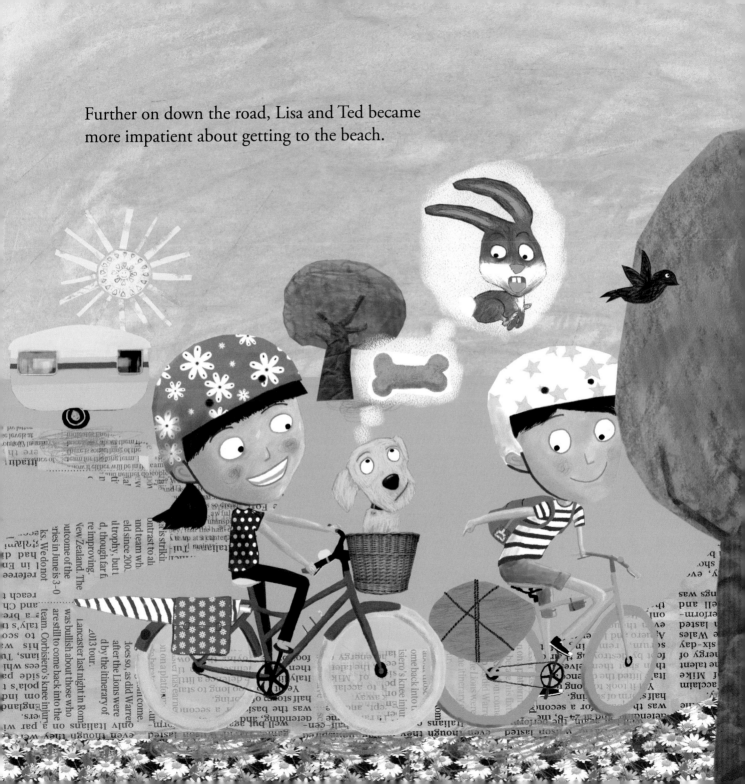

Further on down the road, Lisa and Ted became more impatient about getting to the beach.

My awesome dog nose told me that the beach was not close. I wish Ted's nose had done the same for him because he kept asking, "Are we nearly there?"

"For the last time, when you see the lighthouse we'll nearly be there," Lisa answered, trying to be patient.

"I'm saddle-sore," whined Ted.

"*I'm saddle-sore*," mocked Lisa.

"If you weren't so slow we'd be there by now!" she snapped.

"Humph, well you were the slow one this morning when you couldn't find your swimsuit," muttered Ted. "Well at least I didn't whine like a baby!" teased Lisa.

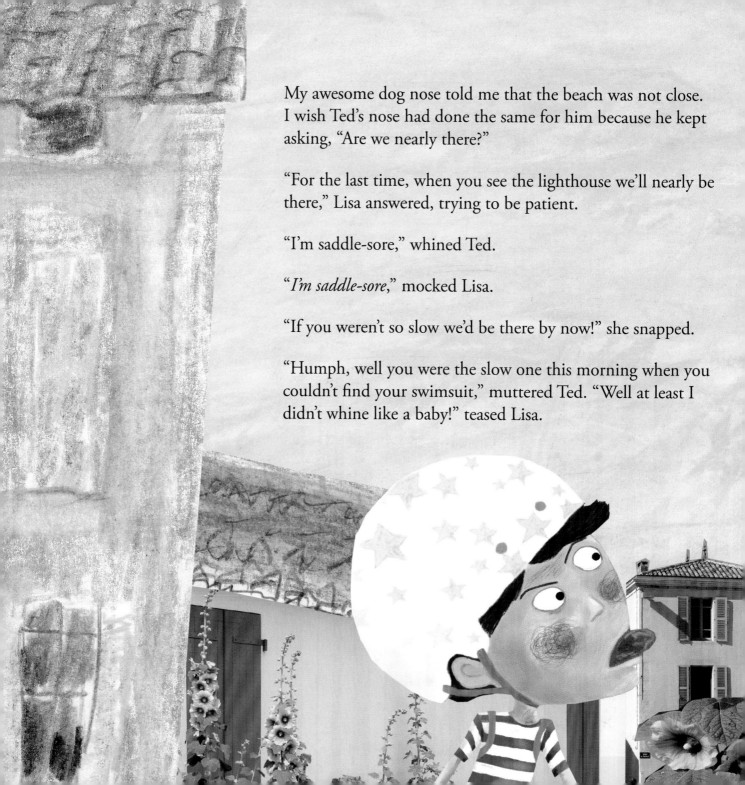

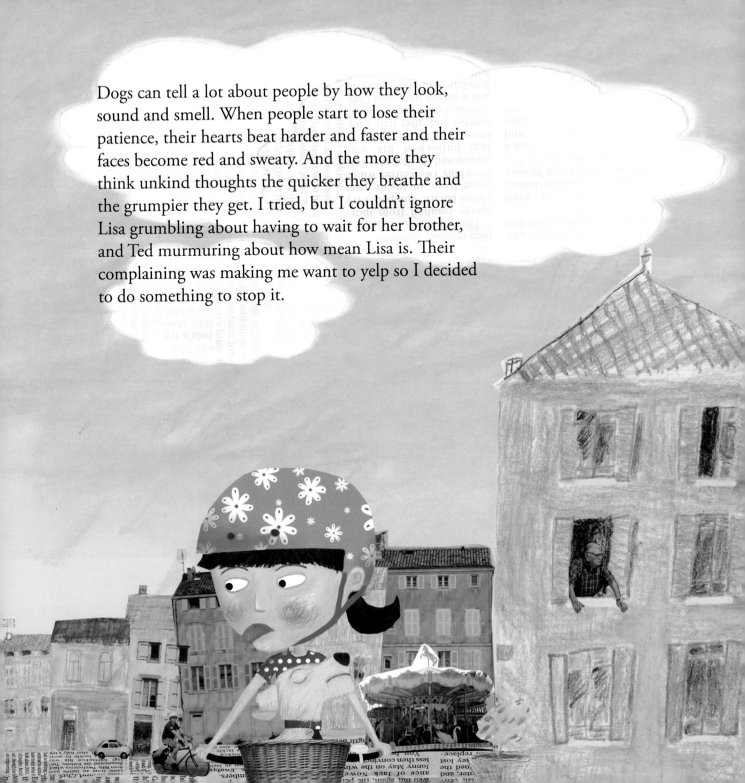

Dogs can tell a lot about people by how they look, sound and smell. When people start to lose their patience, their hearts beat harder and faster and their faces become red and sweaty. And the more they think unkind thoughts the quicker they breathe and the grumpier they get. I tried, but I couldn't ignore Lisa grumbling about having to wait for her brother, and Ted murmuring about how mean Lisa is. Their complaining was making me want to yelp so I decided to do something to stop it.

Staring into Lisa's eyes, with my paw resting on her hand, I thought with all of my might, "Be nice to Ted." Much to my relief, she took a couple of deep breaths and glanced back at her brother. Seeing his tired and unhappy face made her feel bad about being mean to him.

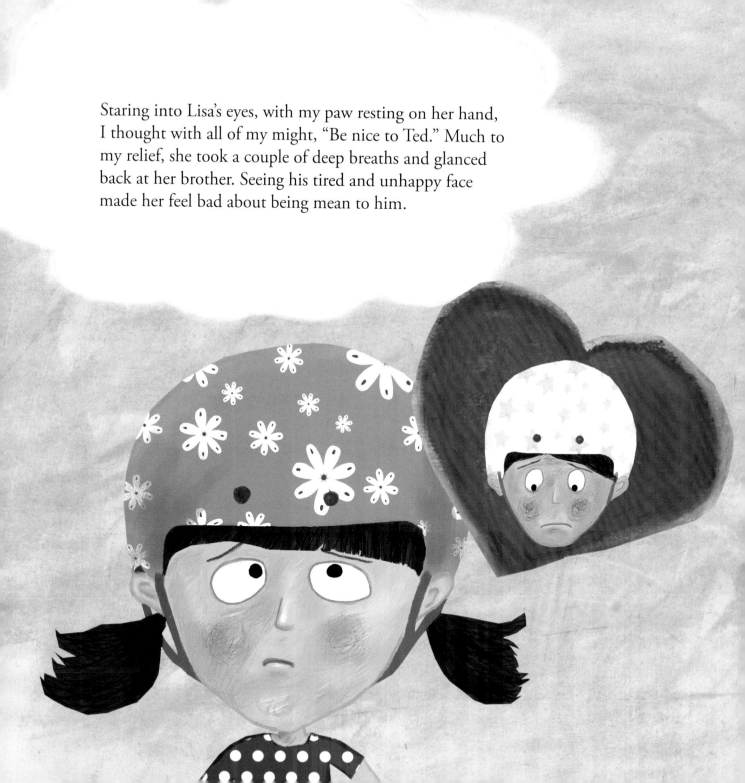

Even though Lisa was still a little annoyed, she stopped and said, "I'm sorry for being mean to you, Ted."

Then, dangling a juicy red strawberry in front of his face, she asked, "Maybe this will make you smile?"

"A doggy biscuit would make me smile!" I barked, but nobody noticed.

"Maybe," muttered Ted, avoiding Lisa's eyes.

"He, he, he, you're trying not to smile," she said, making him laugh. Then, instead of pounding hearts they felt warm and fuzzy inside their chests. Kindness does that to dogs, too, especially when it comes with a belly rub.

"Let's do some Smiling Heart Sounds," Lisa suggested, after they'd had a rest.

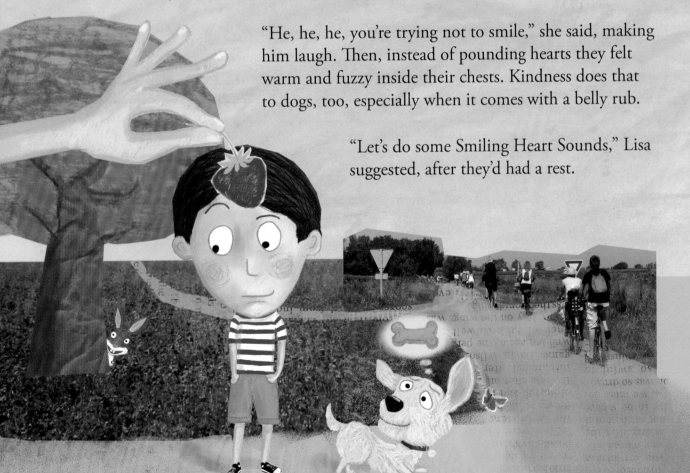

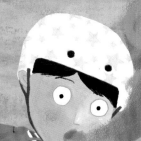

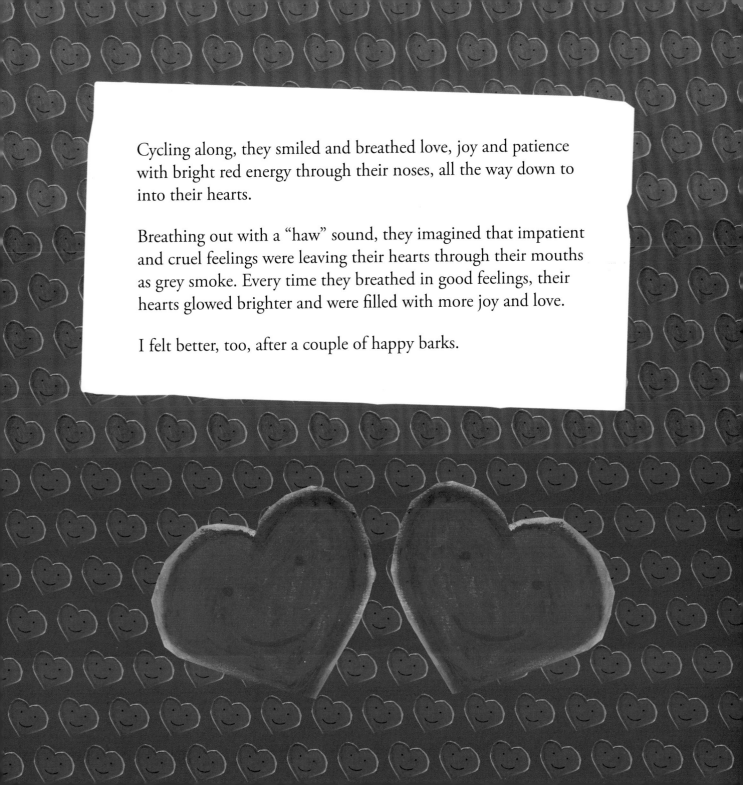

Cycling along, they smiled and breathed love, joy and patience with bright red energy through their noses, all the way down to into their hearts.

Breathing out with a "haw" sound, they imagined that impatient and cruel feelings were leaving their hearts through their mouths as grey smoke. Every time they breathed in good feelings, their hearts glowed brighter and were filled with more joy and love.

I felt better, too, after a couple of happy barks.

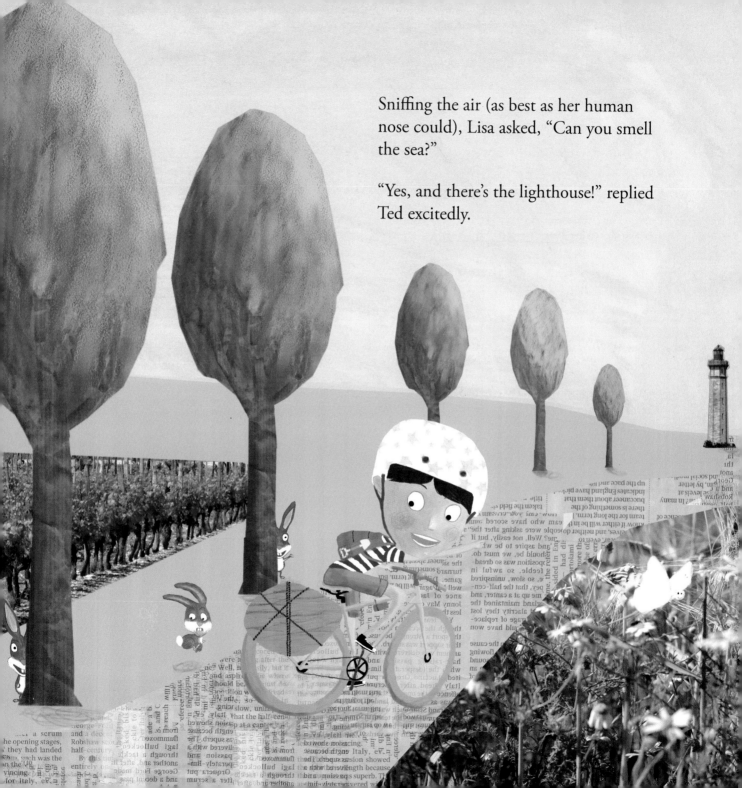

Sniffing the air (as best as her human nose could), Lisa asked, "Can you smell the sea?"

"Yes, and there's the lighthouse!" replied Ted excitedly.

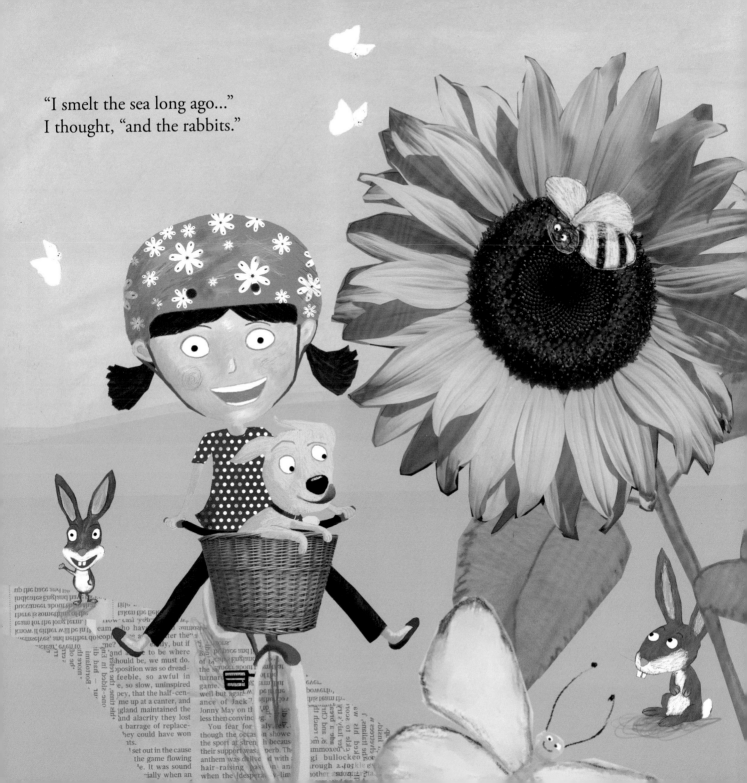

"I smelt the sea long ago..."
I thought, "and the rabbits."

As soon as we got to the beach, I let Lisa know that I was thirsty.

Ted pulled his swimming shorts on and ran off, yelling, "I'm going to be first in! Bring the board when you're coming... please!"

"Okay," replied Lisa, putting a bowl of water down for me.

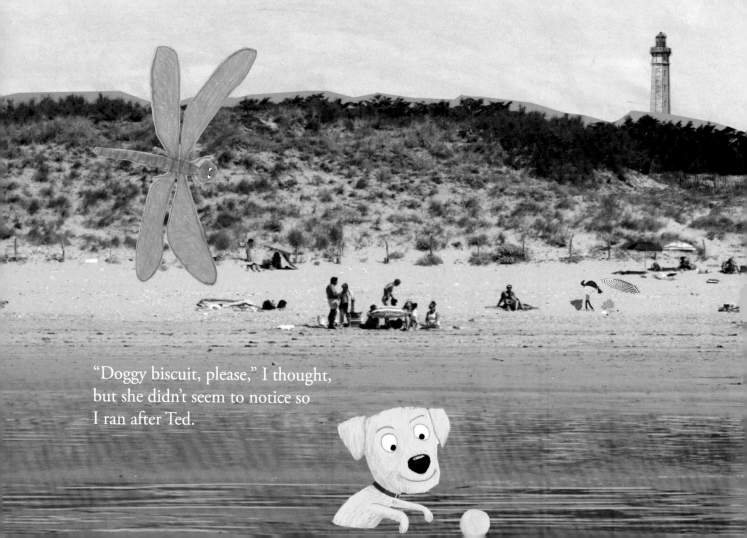

"Doggy biscuit, please," I thought, but she didn't seem to notice so I ran after Ted.

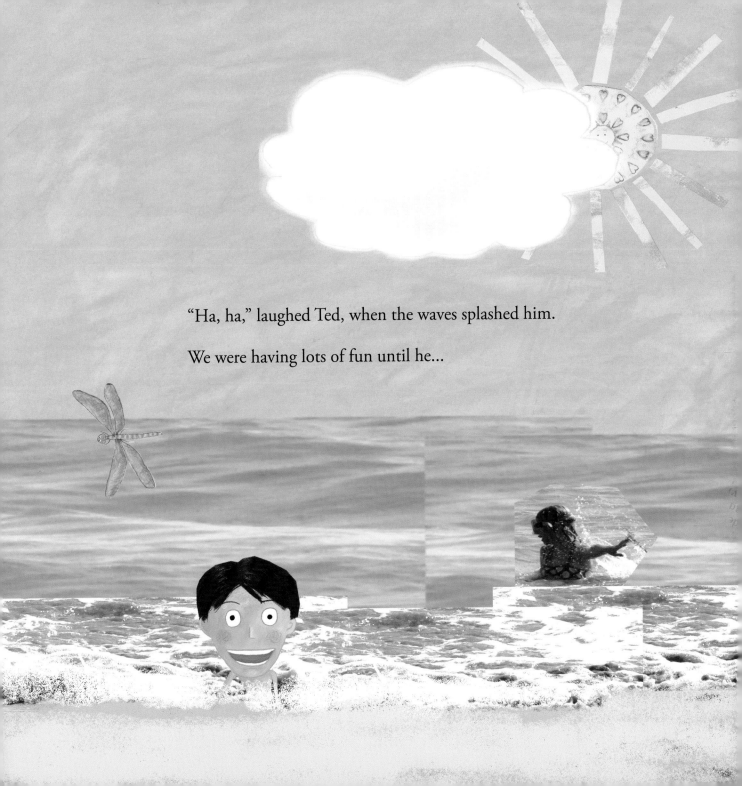

"Ha, ha," laughed Ted, when the waves splashed him.

We were having lots of fun until he...

…looked into the distance to see if Lisa was on her way. "What's taking her so long?" he asked himself, kicking the sand.

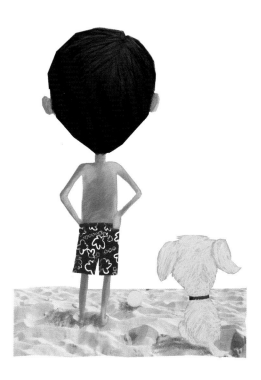

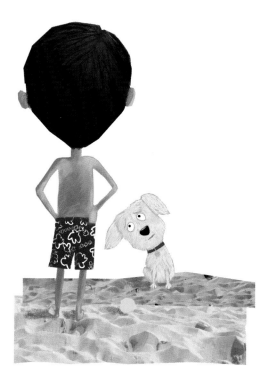

"Never mind, throw the ball again!" I thought, tilting my head to look cute.

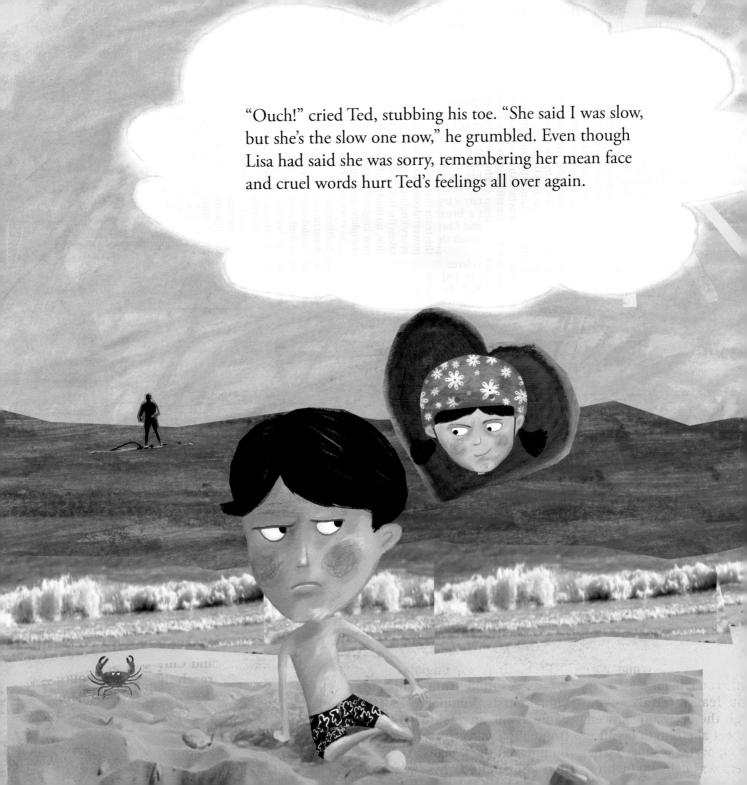

"Ouch!" cried Ted, stubbing his toe. "She said I was slow, but she's the slow one now," he grumbled. Even though Lisa had said she was sorry, remembering her mean face and cruel words hurt Ted's feelings all over again.

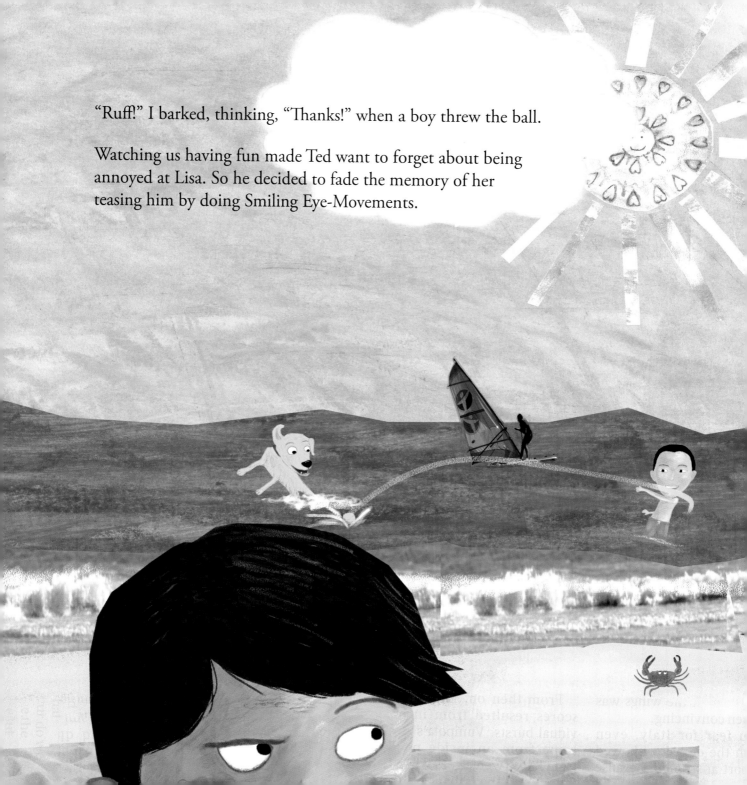

"Ruff!" I barked, thinking, "Thanks!" when a boy threw the ball.

Watching us having fun made Ted want to forget about being annoyed at Lisa. So he decided to fade the memory of her teasing him by doing Smiling Eye-Movements.

Smiling and breathing deeply with his eyes closed, he imagined that he was looking into his heart and seeing Lisa being mean to him.

He breathed deeply into his belly and reminded himself that Lisa is very good to him most of the time.

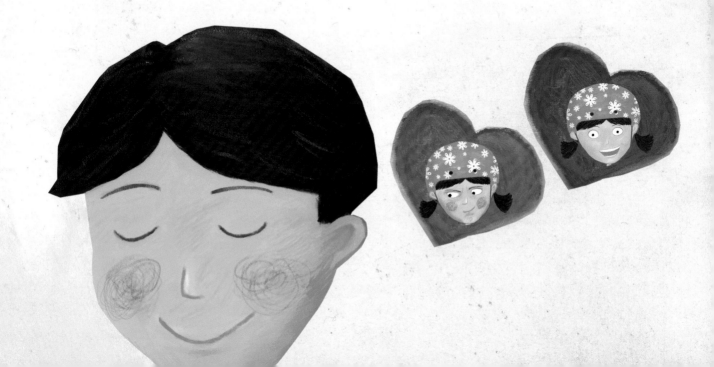

Then, still smiling with his eyes closed, he moved his eyes from left to right ten times. As he did that, Lisa's teasing face slowly faded away, kind of like how the tide washed away my paw prints in the sand.

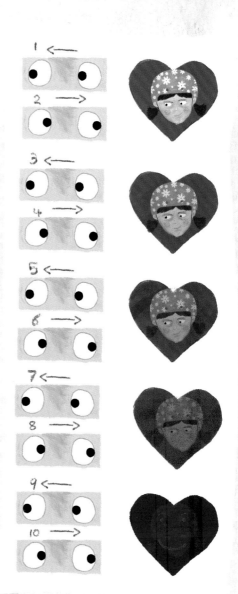

You might think this sounds like
a silly thing to do, but I know it
works. I used to get annoyed when I
remembered the time the neighbour's
dog, Lulu, stole my squeaky toy. But
after I did Smiling Eye-Movements
that memory stopped bothering me
so much.

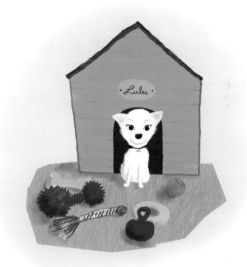

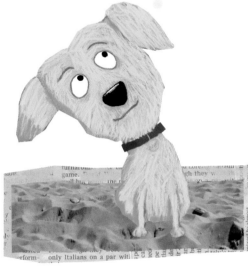

I still growl when she goes
near my toys though.

Smiling with his eyes closed, Ted breathed in love, joy and patience along with red energy into his heart.

"Thank you for trying to protect me, heart. I am fine. Lisa said she was sorry and anyway I could have been kinder to her too. She waits for me a lot and is good at sharing."

Then Ted breathed out his hurt and impatient feelings with a "haw" sound.

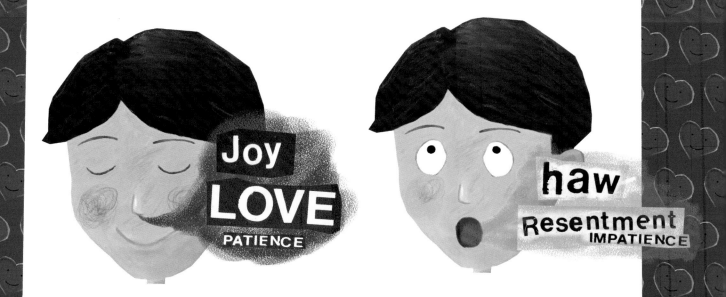

Joy
LOVE
PATIENCE

haw
Resentment
IMPATIENCE

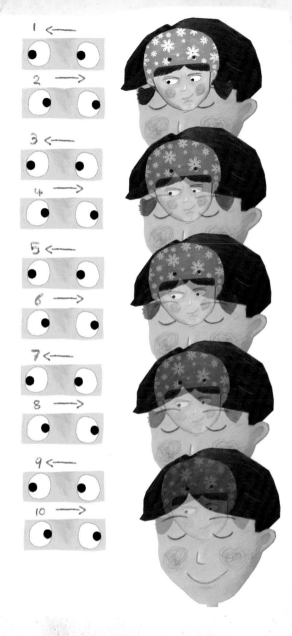

After that his heart felt calmer, but when he closed his eyes he still saw that annoying memory of Lisa very clearly in his head.

So, smiling and keeping his eyes closed, he moved his eyes from left to right ten times and imagined that Lisa's teasing face was fading away from his brain. Once again, he breathed in bright red love into his heart and then breathed out his grumpy feelings with a long, slow "haw" sound.

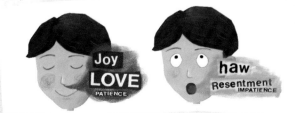

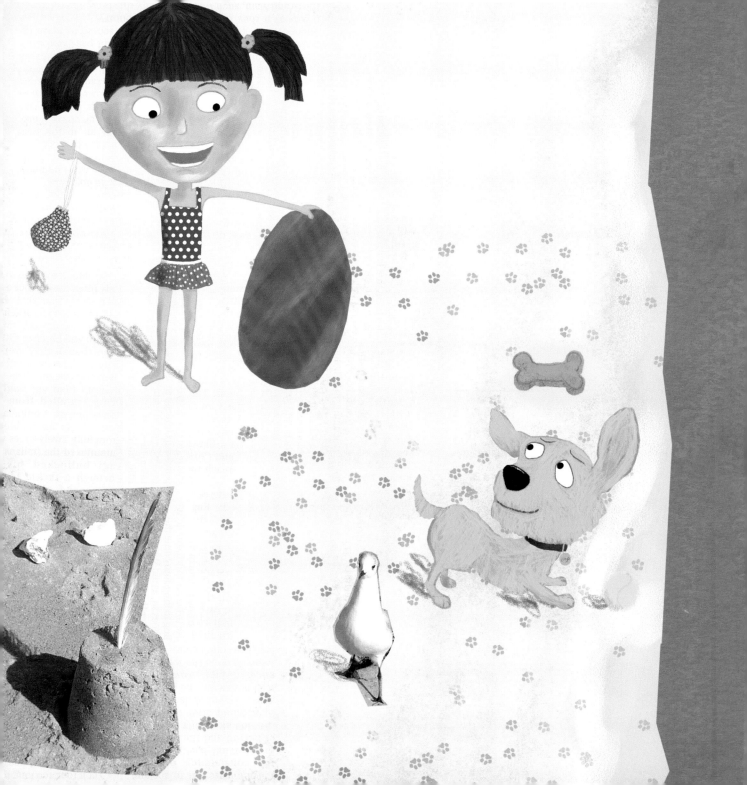

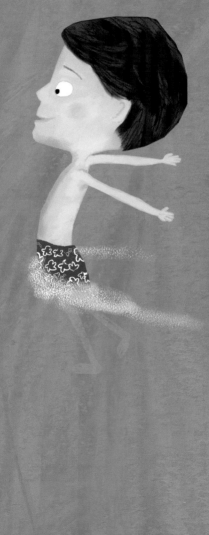

"Yay!" yelled Ted when Lisa came with the board.

I was more excited about the doggy biscuits that I could smell in her bag.

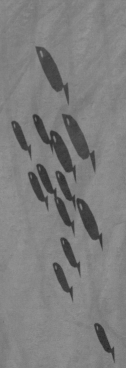

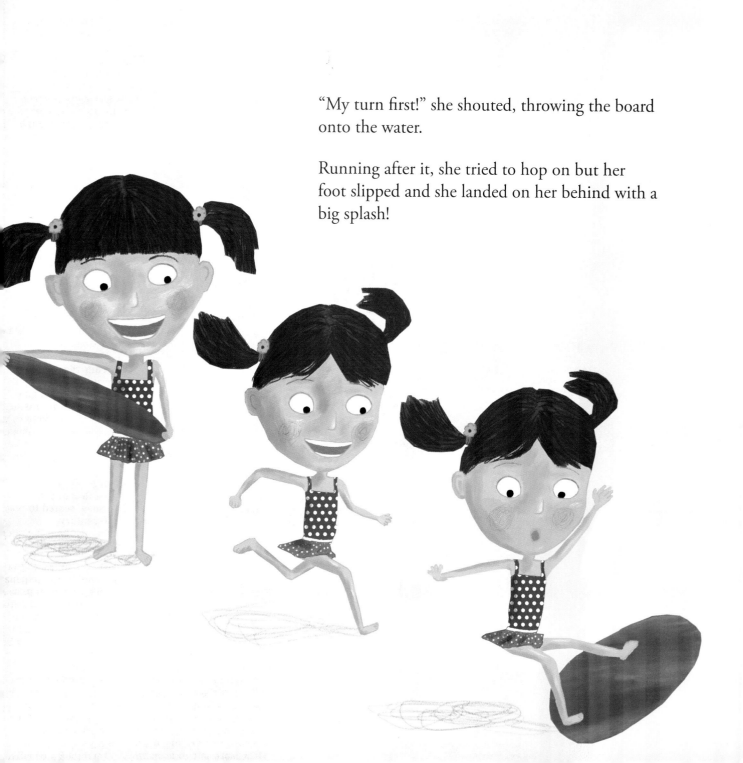

"My turn first!" she shouted, throwing the board onto the water.

Running after it, she tried to hop on but her foot slipped and she landed on her behind with a big splash!

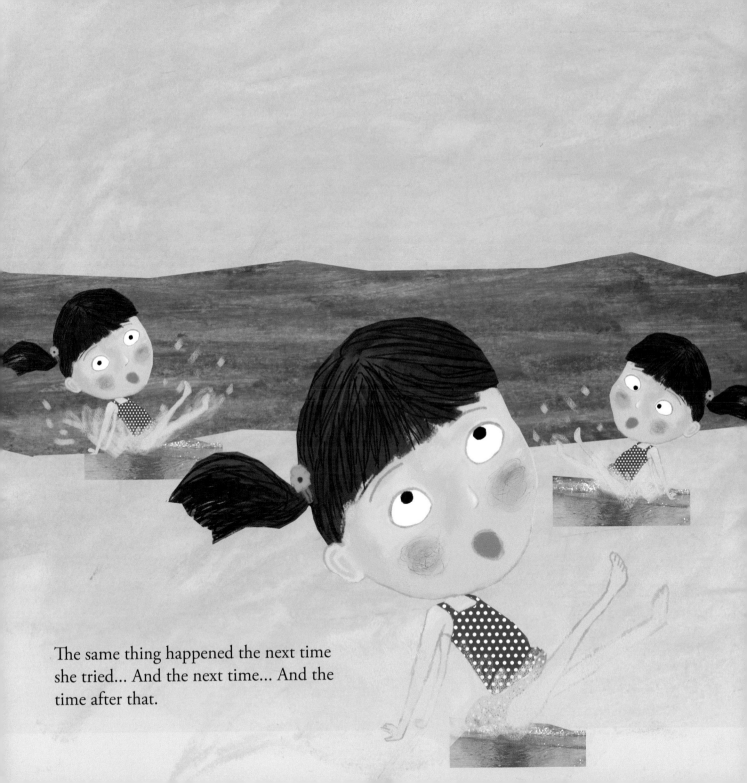

The same thing happened the next time she tried... And the next time... And the time after that.

"Grrr..." growled Lisa, sounding like I do when Lulu's around.

"This is too hard," she whined.

"Keep trying! It's easy peasy, really," said Ted, meaning to be helpful.

Lisa stared at Ted and very slowly said, "I don't want to keep trying."
Then she screamed, "I want to do it now!"

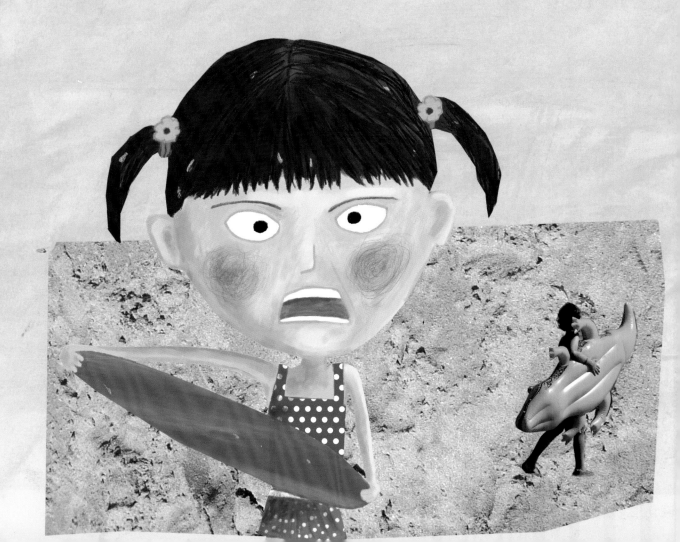

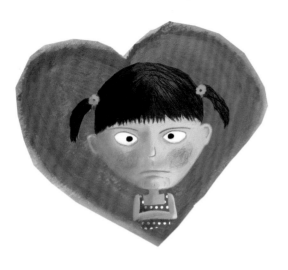

"I'm fed up of trying!" Lisa said, flinging the board down.

Her chin was trembling and she could hardly speak with the lump growing in her throat.

"I'm never going to be able to do that," she mumbled, watching Ted.

I whimpered a little and licked her knee.

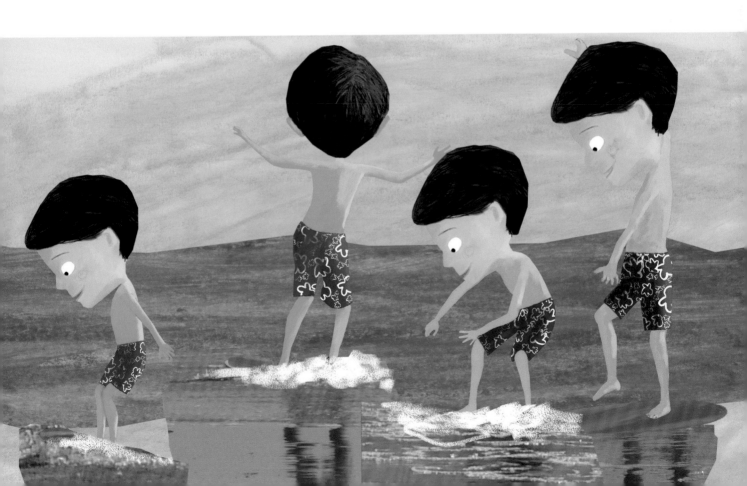

Thankfully, it wasn't long before Lisa got tired of not having fun. She closed her eyes and smiled. Through her nose she breathed in love, joy and patience along with red energy into her heart, while raising her arms above her head.

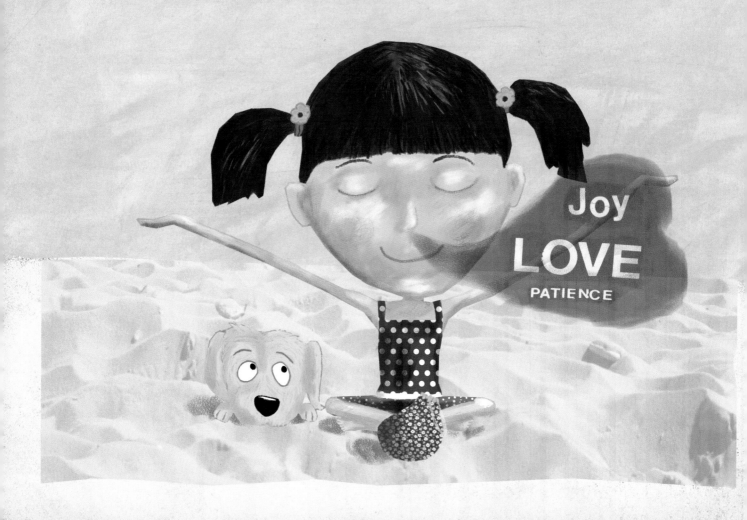

She clasped her hands and turned them upwards so her palms were facing the sky. Then, she looked up, leaned a little to her right and breathed out impatience with a "haw" sound that vibrated inside her heart.

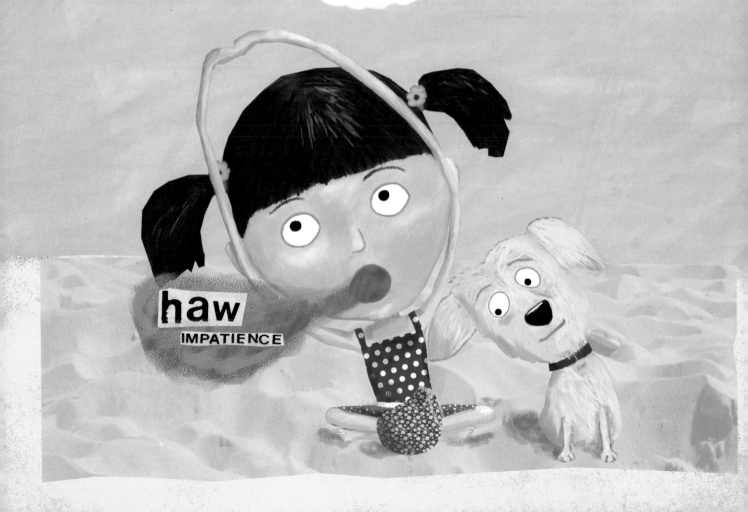

Thinking about how much she loves the summer and playing on the beach with Ted and me, Lisa smiled and gently rubbed her heart.

"Thank you, heart, for pumping my blood and helping me to do things quickly when I need to. It's fine if it takes a while for me to learn how to surf because I'm going to have fun trying," she whispered.

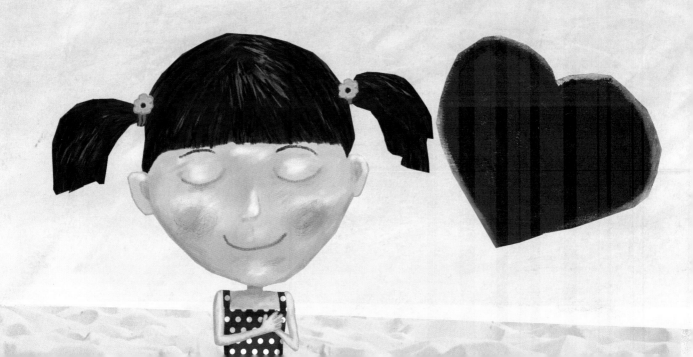

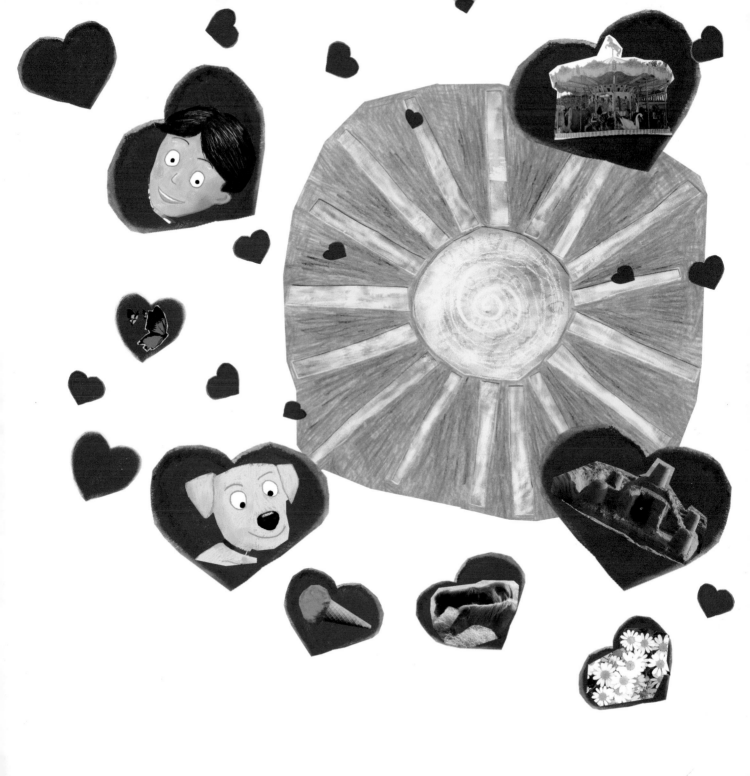

Feeling calmer, Lisa stood up and wiped
the sand off herself.

Picking up the board, she gave me a little wink
and then said to Ted, "Right, stand back and
watch the expert!"

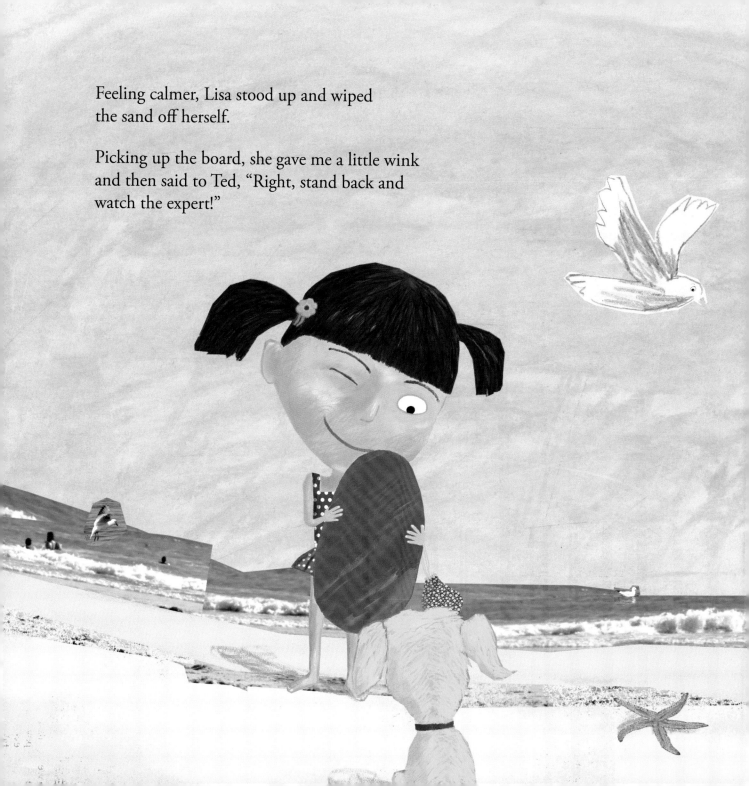

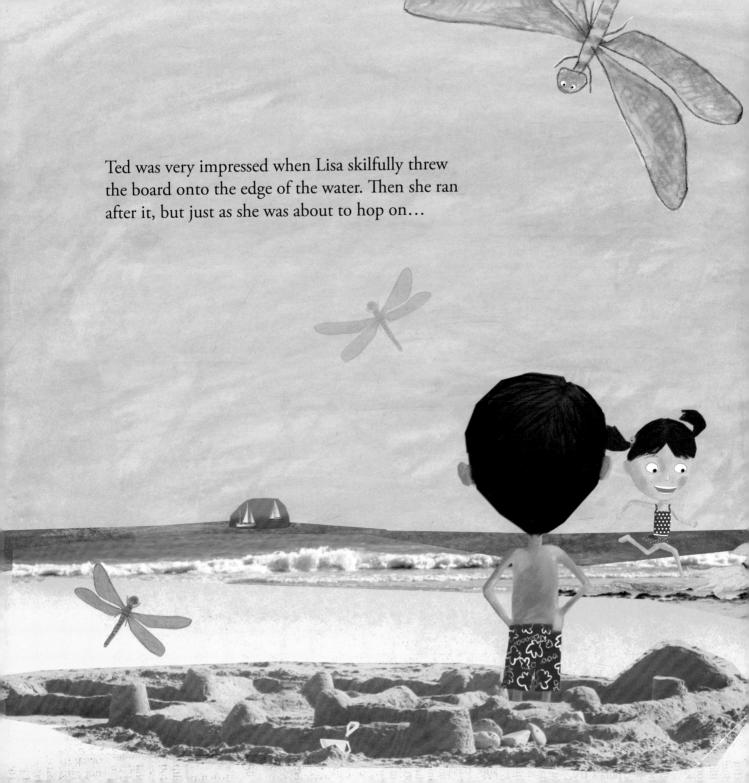

Ted was very impressed when Lisa skilfully threw
the board onto the edge of the water. Then she ran
after it, but just as she was about to hop on…

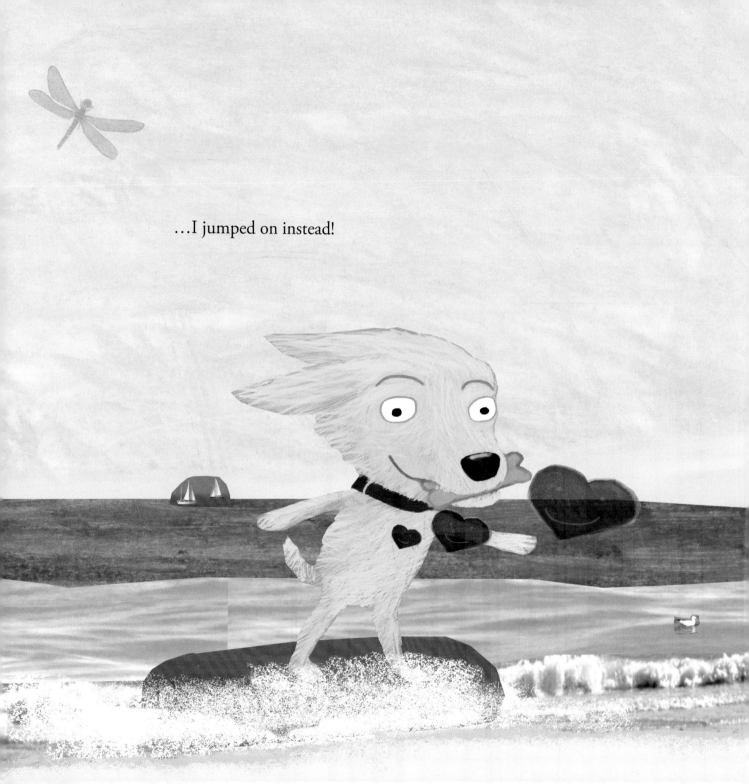

...I jumped on instead!

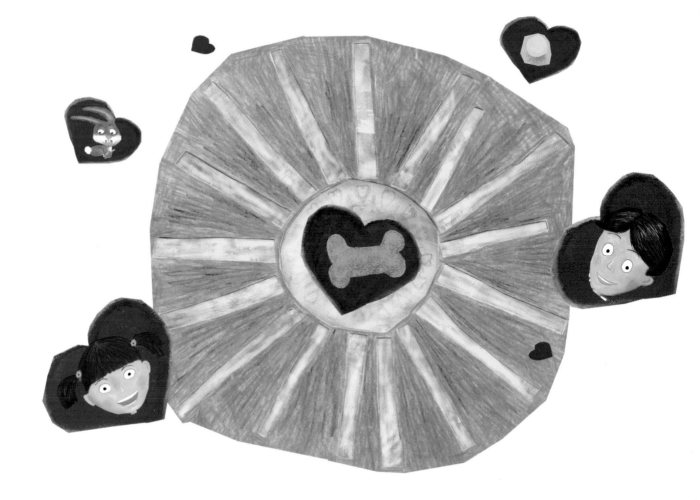

"Ha, ha, ha… Clever dog, Bingo! That's just what
I wanted you to do! You read my mind!" yelled Lisa,
tossing me a doggy biscuit.

"And, at last, you read mine too," I thought,
munching happily.

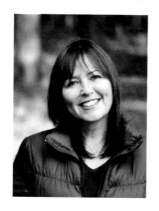

About the Author

Lisa Spillane qualified as a teacher of Art and Design at NCAD in Dublin, Ireland. She has a Master's degree in Education and is a co-founder and former Director of Artlink Ltd., a charitable company promoting access to art in the north west of Ireland. Having taught at a number of schools, Lisa went on to work for several years in Northern Ireland for NIACRO on community projects with children and young people. She learned Qigong meditation from attending classes taught by Grandmaster Mantak Chia. Lisa has recently moved to England from Brussels, Belgium.

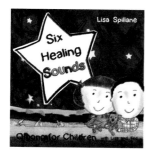

Also by Lisa Spillane...

Six Healing Sounds with Lisa and Ted
Qigong for Children
ISBN 978 1 84819 051 1
eISBN 978 0 85701 031 5

Six Healing Sounds with Lisa and Ted teaches young children how to transform negative feelings into positive ones by using simple breathing techniques that are based on ancient Chinese Qigong exercises. Using a special sound for different parts of the body, Lisa and Ted show that a "haaaww" can heal the heart and blow away impatience, and a "whooooooo" can steady the stomach and chase away worries. These reassuring meditative stories are ideal for bedtime as they calm and settle children by soothing away the troubles of the day.

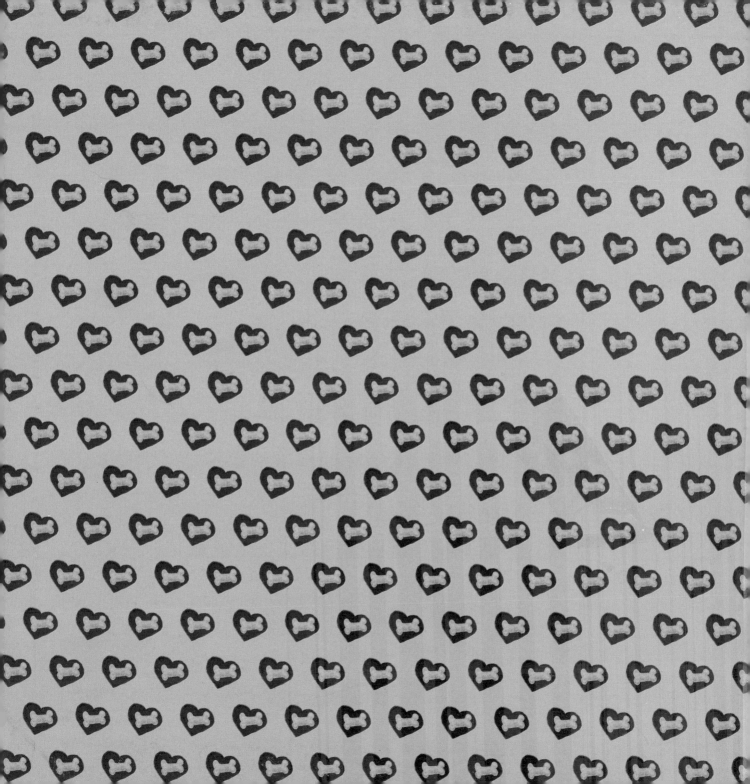